Sue Says: Mantras To Love Yourself Forever Thin

by Sue Yelvington

Sue Yelvington
Published by: Main Street Digi
4435 N First Street #191
Livermore CA 94550
jeanne@mainstreetdigi.com

The author welcomes
your comments and suggestions

Forward

Mantras are a word or a phrase that are repeated often or that expresses someone's basic beliefs. Mantras have been life changing for me.

I started using them as a young mother beginning to build my first business from my home. I was scared and unsure of myself. I had so much to learn and I felt I was really sticking my neck out.

No one among my family and friends thought I should begin my own business. Almost everyone tried to talk me out of it. I just had a deep knowing that this was the right path and took the plunge anyway.

It took a lot of courage for me to put myself out in the world as a beginning business woman, especially with no real support.

I had only been married a year and a half. I had a six-month old baby and I was learning to be a step mom as well. I was also stepping into the world of business as someone who'd only worked in jobs where the duties were clear cut and repetitive.

I had high hopes in the beginning and was unprepared for the learning curve. There was so much I had to learn about business, attitude, focus, and follow through, and so much more. As it turned out, starting that business was one of the best educational adventures of my life.

Eventually I learned that whenever I faced fears and other challenges, I would set my mind on some new goal or skill I needed to learn. Then I would develop a mantra that was easy to say and remember.

If not me, who? If not now, when? I'd focus on that mantra and skill until I mastered what I was trying to accomplish. Then I'd set a new goal, find a new mantra and onward and upward I went.

I continue to use mantras in every area of my life to this day. They're easy to remember and they keep me on track. I share these with you to not only help you shed weight and get healthy, but to help you in other areas of your life as well.

My suggestion is that you
- choose the mantra that best suits your needs and challenges at that particular time.
- put it where you can see it easily and regularly.

You might even write your mantra on file cards or post it notes and put then all around your house, office, or even your car.

It won't take long and the mantra will come to mind easily. You'll be surprised how much mantras can help you transform your life and habits!

I wish you joy and celebration as you master the skills necessary to drop weight and create the life of your dreams!

All the BEST!
Sue

When I know better, I'll do better.

Everyone, including you, is doing the best they can. No one sets out to do a bad job. The truth is you are doing the best you can with what you have to work with. In fact, if you look back on what you classify as mistakes AND take into consideration the time, money, energy and knowledge that you had back then, you'll see that it's the only decision you could have made. If you want to do better, you need to improve what you're already doing or learn something new. Little by little you can improve. There's no point in beating yourself up for doing not doing better. So just remember when you know better, you'll do better.

As I learn to truly love myself, the weight will melt off.

Love is such a powerful force!   I'm talking about unconditional love.   Everyone we love has traits that could be perceived as flaws, and we love them anyway. Love yourself flaws and all!   As you do, pay attention to what makes you feel good, and you'll want to do more of that. Explore what foods are really satisfying to you, savor each delicious bite, notice what foods give you energy. Love the food, love your body, love yourself.

I put my own oxygen mask on first.

When the flight attendant is presenting the air flight safety instructions, you are told to put your own oxygen mask on before you help others with theirs. What's the reason for that? If you run out of air, you're not capable of helping anyone with anything. What this really means is your self-care must be your top priority. It's a top priority because otherwise you don't have the energy, the mood, the thought process, the patience to do what you need and want to do for others. Remember, self-care is your oxygen mask

Happiness is an inside job.

Abe Lincoln said, people are about as happy as they decide to be. It's a fact, we each make our own happiness. It does not come from outside of us. I'll bet there have been times when you heard someone complain about something that you would have been thrilled to experience. You want to start developing the ability to be happy with every experience. Count your blessings and find the gift in every situation. A good situation will bring out the happiness that's already inside of you. You'll find that you'll get happier and happier. When you're happy, you do better! You might even want to start a gratitude journal. Recording all the blessings in your life, big and small, will increase your happiness very quickly!

To thine own self be true.

Are you aware that everybody's finger prints are different and unique? That is because we are each unique right down to our fingerprints. And, yet as humans, we try to be like everybody else so that we fit in. We are afraid that if we are too different we will be excluded. The truth is that when you get comfortable with the truth of who you are and live from that, you will draw people to you who appreciate what you offer. More importantly, when you experience yourself as enough and appreciate the uniqueness of you, you will be happier; more fulfilled and bring more of yourself into expression. You will become happier and happier.

What am I really hungry for?

Ask yourself this question when you start to reach for some food or drink that is not part of your healthy food plan. Often people reach for food when they are really thirsty. Different emotions can drive us to eat different foods. Crunchy food when you're angry, comfort food when you're sad, sweets when you feel very depressed, etc. Pause for a few minutes, get quiet and ask yourself, what am I hungry for?

My health is my greatest wealth.

It's absolutely true! If you don't feel well, if you're achy and tired, there's a good chance that you are not living the life of your dreams. We all have dreams and goals inside of us. Often when we don't feel well, when we're tired, and achy due to ailments or simply being overweight--we lose track of those dreams. People will sometimes complain that they're too tired to play with their kids or grandkids. They have stopped doing the things they used to like to do. They often feel like a disappointment to themselves. That's certainly poverty thinking! It doesn't have to be that way. You can be rich in mind, body and soul by improving your health conditions. Change what you eat, what you do, and how you think and you'll live a richer life.

I choose to be slim, healthy, and full of life.

It's a powerful affirmation. One important thing to notice is that you're not saying, "I *want* to be ..." "I want" creates a state of emptiness that people often try to fill up with substances and activities. That might work for the moment, but the results are not lasting. Using the words "I choose" or "I decide" creates a much stronger and loving statement. It comes from being responsible for your well being and sense of worth. Let me caution you, don't just say the words like a robot, that won't work. Create positive emotion, see the slim healthy you, and feel how that would feel! It takes practice. It's not a huge effort and the payoff is life changing!

When I eat better, I feel better.

You know that's the truth. You might start looking at yourself like you're a science or a chemistry experiment. Pay attention to how you feel when you eat certain things and what you eat at various times. Often carbs like pancakes, bread, and grains create a short-lived sugar spike that gets you going but then drops you into a low blood sugar fog. So, you reach for more sugar or caffeine to get an energy boost and the vicious cycle continues. Make a game out of learning what works for you and what doesn't.

When I look better, I feel better.

Sometimes we lose track of the little things that make us look and feel better. We wear clothes even though we feel unattractive in them. We squeeze into clothes that create bulges and feel too tight. We don't buy new clothes because we're going to lose weight first. However, when we don't feel attractive, we are more likely to overeat or make poor food choices. So, don't punish yourself. Find or buy clothes that make you feel good and look good too. Take care of your hair, makeup, hygiene, and whatever else makes you feel beautiful, cared for, and uniquely you!

There's a reason the word die is in the word diet.

Most diets don't work and they often undermine one's health. The majority of people who lose weight on a diet gain all of it back and then some. When you starve your body and then turn around and over feed it, you are abusing it. Those diets are doomed to fail. What you really want to do is create better habits which will create a healthy lifestyle that will keep you slim. When you really have a healthy plan, you'll drop weight fairly quickly. Stick to it long enough, it becomes a habit. Bottom line: if you want to sustain your ideal weight, you must have a lifestyle that supports it.

A habit is simply
a repetitive behavior.

It's a behavior pattern that you've followed so long and so often that now it's almost involuntary. You've been doing it so long that when you don't do it, your body gets uncomfortable and it stirs up emotion. You can't just drop a habit. You want to replace it with a new behavior that supports your new healthy goals. Use your imagination.

You might want to make a list of things to try and work with them each for a few days until you find the thing that will support you changing your old habit. When you find the ideas you like best, use it for 21 days. It's been long said that it takes 21 days to create a habit.

A belief is just a thought you keep thinking.

We are given rules to live by. We're taught many ways of thinking and viewing the world. When we're little, we have no filter, so these beliefs get planted within us. We then live by these beliefs without questioning them. History has shown us that many accepted beliefs change as new information comes to light. A wise person questions these beliefs and discovers if they are really true. As you release outdated beliefs and create new, uplifting beliefs, you'll see your life change dramatically.

Nothing tastes as good
as thin feels.

When you're reaching for that bag of cookies, or that chocolate remember this! That momentary pleasure is not going to get you to your goal. When you're faced with a trigger food, if you say this mantra to yourself, it can often get you to stop long enough that you won't eat it.

Cravings are my body's call for better nutrition.

Your cravings are your body's way to tell you what it needs. For instance, craving chocolate is often a signal that you need more magnesium. There are charts you can find online that will suggest what the craving is really trying to tell you. When the cells in your body have the nutrition they need, they're happy and healthy. You'll have a lot more energy. Your cravings will change and you'll want healthy food. Get the nutrition that you need and watch those cravings just go away.

Food won't fill an emotional need.

There are so many variations on what we eat, drink, or do to try to escape our emotions. If you don't deal with the emotions that are causing you to overeat or eat the wrong things, you're never going to win the battle. These emotions block our joy, our creativity, even our ability to love whole heartedly. When we face our fears, our unruly emotions, we begin to feel whole, happy, and at peace. Pay attention to those emotions without judgment. Heal your emotions and watch your food cravings go away.

A minute on the lips, a year on the hips.

It's a momentary pleasure, that really isn't a pleasure because pretty soon you begin to feel guilty. "I'll just have one brownie. Well I'll just have one more." Then you ate the whole pan. Pretty soon, you're down that slippery slope of self-loathing, guilt, and hopelessness. Was it really worth it?

Sugar is the root of all evil.

Sugar causes inflammation. Sugar causes cravings. Sugar can cause anxiety. If your blood sugar shoots up and drops down rapidly, it can put you an emotional roller coaster. I use the term sugar loosely. I also mean things like pasta, rice, bread, and foods that quickly metabolize and give you a rush, a sugar high. These days we have super sugar, high fructose corn syrup. Fake food manufacturers are putting sugar in everything. Be aware, read labels. If it ends in "-ose", it's sugar: glucose, fructose, dextrose, etc. You can search online and get a list. Avoid them like the plague, cut them out!

If the food is in a box,
it's not food.

It's processed nothing. You might as well eat the cardboard box it came in. There's no real nutrition in most of it. When you eat it, you might be full for a while, and then you'll have cravings and be hungry because your cells aren't being fed. Eventually, you're going to eat more because your body will drive you to it. This is why we overeat. Eat real food and you'll eat less and be more satisfied.

Thank you belly,
for holding my emotions
I wasn't yet ready to deal with.

The seat of your emotions is in your middle area and that's where so many of us carry excess weight. It's a protective padding. Instead of being angry at your body for having a big belly, thank it for finding a way to protect you from having to feel the emotions you weren't yet ready to release and process. As you work through the emotions you've been stuffing, you'll find yourself with a slimmer middle.

I'm not deprived, I'm investing in my future health and wellbeing.

As we start eliminating foods and things that we are used to eating, it's common for people to feel deprived. As you begin to feel and look better, as the excess weight drops off, you aren't going to feel deprived. You'll find that you don't like those old, unhealthy foods anymore. You won't feel deprived because you won't like them anymore.

Don't go to a party
with an empty stomach.

Parties can be dangerous to your food plan. If you're hungry, you may end up eating the wrong foods and too much of them. So, eat before you go to a party. When you're at the party, savor small bites that give you a taste and don't throw you totally off your plan. Another idea is to bring something that's on your plan to the party which ensures there is at least one thing you can eat.

Emotions are simply signals.

Our bodies, our spirits are trying to communicate with us. Here's how it works...we have a thought, and based on our conditioning, the thought creates an emotion. The emotion shows up as a feeling in our body, like butterflies in our stomach or a headache. If we associate that feeling with something painful, we often don't want to face it or relive it. So, we stuff it down or find some way to avoid feeling it. That keeps the feeling stuck in our body, acting on us in ways that don't serve our highest interest. Here's a simple way to honor our feelings and allow them to dissipate. Recognize where in your body an emotion is showing up, and send that emotion love. Do it until you feel the emotion shift. It may lighten up, it may go away. You might feel the emotion shift and change to different emotions in different places in your body. Just follow each emotion without judgment and send it love. It will eventually be healed.

Conclusion

It is my strong desire that the mantras in this book served to help you discover and transform some of your previous limiting beliefs into beliefs that support you in dropping weight and living a happy life. I also hope that you recognize that changing your life can be as simple (and as difficult) as changing your mind.

We live in an ever-expanding universe. If you want to feel more connected to yourself, more in tune with life; then getting your thoughts and energy in alignment is key. There are times when a mirror reflecting our thoughts and beliefs back to us can be very useful. As a coach, I have been that mirror for many people. If that resonates with you and you'd like to explore it, please reach out.

I help people get more clarity about their weight issues, I would love to offer you a free coaching session as my schedule allows. First you complete a survey that I will send to you, then we can schedule the session.. In this session we identify your goals, challenges, and ways you might be self-sabotaging. We often begin to formulate a plan to help you achieve the Forever Thin Body of your dreams!

You can contact me me via Facebook by searching for Sue Yelvington. You can also contact me by email. My email is: sue@sueyelvington.com.

If you'd like to access the Forever Thin free coaching session, just reach out. First you receive a survey, then we can schedule your session.

I'd love to hear from you

Facebook: Sue Yelvington

Email: sue@sueyelvington.com

!

www.ingramcontent.com/pod-product-compliance
Lightning Source LLC
Chambersburg PA
CBHW061946280526
45787CB00004B/1737